CAYENNE PEPPER DIET

A Comprehensive Guide to the Cayenne Pepper Diet and its Benefits

Anthony Malachy

TABLE OF CONTENT

CHAPTER ONE
Introduction.

The 10-day cayenne pepper diet, sometimes referred to as the Master Cleanse or Lemonade Diet, encourages consumption of a concoction of water, lemon juice, maple syrup, and cayenne pepper. Although some individuals assert that the diet provides a number of advantages, there isn't any scientific proof to back up these assertions. The following are some alleged advantages of the cayenne pepper diet:

The cayenne pepper diet is said to aid in detoxification by removing waste products and toxins from the body.

Loss of weight: Because the diet severely restricts calories, it may cause fast weight loss.

Improved digestion: It is said that include lemon juice in your diet may help with bloating and constipation as well as improve digestion.

Energy boost: Some dieters claim to feel more energised and alert, probably as a result of the caffeine and other ingredients in cayenne pepper.

Reduced inflammation: The anti-inflammatory chemical capsaicin, which is present in cayenne pepper, may aid in reducing inflammation in the body.

But it's important to remember that there isn't much scientific proof to back up many of these advantages. The cayenne pepper diet is also unsustainable and unhealthy over the long run since it has very few calories and inadequate nourishment. The diet should not be followed by anybody who has specific medical issues, such as diabetes or renal disease. It is always advisable to speak with a healthcare practitioner before beginning any detoxification or weight-loss program to identify the best course of action for your particular requirements.

How the cayenne pepper diet works:

The cayenne pepper diet, sometimes referred to as the Master Cleanse or Lemonade Diet, promotes the body's detoxification and calorie restriction states. For ten days, participants on the diet ingest a concoction comprising water, cayenne pepper, maple syrup, and lemon juice. The diet functions as follows:

Calorie restriction: The cayenne pepper diet offers just 600–1200 calories per day, which is quite little calories. The body is forced to utilize fat reserves for energy as a consequence of the extreme calorie restriction, which may cause fast weight loss.

By removing waste materials and toxins from the body, the diet is thought to aid in detoxification. According to legend, the cayenne pepper and lemon juice in the combination stimulate the liver and help in toxin removal via the urine and feces.

Appetite suppression: Some dieters claim to feel less hungry, presumably as a result of the appetite-suppressing properties of cayenne pepper.

Increased metabolism: The chemical capsaicin, which is present in cayenne pepper, is thought to speed up the body's metabolism and encourage the burning of fat.

Better digestion: It is said that the lemon juice in the dish can help digestion and ease bloating and constipation.

Although the cayenne pepper diet is incredibly low in calories and does not give enough nourishment, it is important to note that it is not a long-term eating strategy that is healthful or sustainable. In addition, the weight reduction seen while on the diet can be attributable to a loss of water and muscle mass rather than fat, and it might be restored after returning to regular eating. It is not advised to follow the cayenne pepper diet in order to lose weight permanently or to address health issues.

The History of Cayenne Pepper:

Red pepper, commonly referred to as cayenne pepper, has been a staple ingredient in many different cuisines for thousands of years. Cayenne pepper has a long history, and both the Americas and Europe have produced proof of its usage.

The Capsicum annuum plant, which is indigenous to Central and South America, is the source of cayenne pepper. It is well known that the ancient Mayans and Aztecs cultivated and used a variety of chili peppers, including cayenne, in their cuisine. These civilizations also employed cayenne pepper in traditional medicine because they thought it had healing qualities including pain alleviation and digestive help.

Cayenne pepper was brought to other regions of the globe with the advent of Europeans in the Americas in the 15th and 16th century. It swiftly gained popularity in Europe, where it was utilized as a cheaper alternative to pricey and challenging-to-find black pepper at the time. Cayenne pepper was initially brought to India by the Portuguese, where it was well-received and utilized in a variety of recipes.

The Spanish brought cayenne pepper to America for the first time in the sixteenth century. It gained popularity in Southern cooking swiftly, where it was used to spice up and flavor meals like gumbo and jambalaya.

Cayenne pepper is a common ingredient in many different dishes nowadays and is renowned for its intense heat and distinctive taste. It is also used in conventional medicine and is thought to provide a number of health advantages, including better digestion and increased metabolism. Many well-known spicy sauces, like Tabasco sauce, have cayenne pepper as a primary component.

How cayenne pepper was used in ancient medicine:

Many ancient societies have utilized cayenne pepper (Capsicum annuum), which has a long history of usage in traditional medicine, for a variety of therapeutic reasons. Here are a few instances of the ancient uses for cayenne pepper in medicine:

Relief from pain: The active component of cayenne pepper, capsaicin, is a natural painkiller. It is thought that endorphins, the body's natural painkillers, may be released in response to the heat from capsaicin. Cayenne pepper was utilized by ancient doctors to treat arthritis, headaches, and toothaches.

Cayenne pepper was utilized as a digestive remedy to enhance digestion and ease gastrointestinal problems including constipation, bloating, and gas. The synthesis of digestive enzymes may be stimulated and blood flow to the digestive system may be increased by the cayenne pepper's heat, according to some theories.

Anti-inflammatory: Rheumatoid arthritis, bronchitis, and sore throats have all been treated with cayenne pepper as an anti-inflammatory. Ancient healers employed cayenne pepper to help lessen inflammation and advance healing since capsaicin has been demonstrated to have anti-inflammatory effects.

Support for the circulatory system: Cayenne pepper was utilized to encourage normal blood flow and enhance circulation. Cayenne pepper was thought to be able to decrease blood pressure, lower cholesterol, and prevent blood clots.

Overall, cayenne pepper was valued as a therapeutic plant in many ancient societies, and contemporary research has validated its numerous use in traditional medicine. Cayenne pepper may irritate the digestive system in big doses, and it can even harm it, so it's crucial to use it sensibly and under a doctor's supervision.

CHAPTER TWO
The science behind the cayenne pepper diet.

The cayenne pepper diet, commonly referred to as the Master Cleanse, is a kind of detoxification that calls for ingesting a concoction of cayenne pepper, lemon juice, maple syrup, and water over the course of 10 to 14 days. The diet's proponents claim that it may aid in promoting weight reduction, enhancing digestion, and detoxifying the body. There is, however, little solid scientific proof to back up these assertions.

Because it contains capsaicin, a substance that may aid in

boosting metabolism and promoting weight reduction, cayenne pepper is thought to be a crucial component of the cayenne pepper diet. According to some research, capsaicin may enhance calorie burning by boosting fat oxidation and energy expenditure. Capsaicin does have a little impact on weight reduction, thus it could not be substantial enough to provide appreciable outcomes.

Additionally, it is said that the cayenne pepper diet aids in cleansing and betters digestion. These assertions are, however, not well supported by science. While the cayenne pepper diet's high calorie restriction may be harmful and may cause vitamin shortages, muscle loss, and a slower metabolism, lemon juice and maple syrup can assist offer some nutrients and energy throughout the diet.

The cayenne pepper diet is also not a healthy or sustainable approach to lose weight and improve your health over the long run. Numerous detrimental health consequences, such as exhaustion, lightheadedness, headaches, and electrolyte imbalances, might result from the high calorie restriction and absence of a well-balanced diet.

Overall, the cayenne pepper diet is not a scientifically supported or safe way to lose weight or improve general health, despite the fact that cayenne pepper may have some possible health advantages. Before beginning any kind of severe diet or detox program, it is crucial to talk with a healthcare provider.

How cayenne pepper helps with weight loss and detoxification:

Capsaicin, a chemical found in cayenne pepper, a kind of chili pepper, has been demonstrated to offer a number of health advantages, including detoxification and weight reduction.

Cayenne pepper may help with detoxification and weight reduction in the following ways:

Boosts metabolism: Studies have indicated that the cayenne pepper's capsaicin increases energy expenditure and metabolism, which may aid in calorie burning and weight reduction.

Reduces hunger and increases feelings of fullness, which may help individuals eat fewer calories and lose weight. Cayenne pepper may help suppress appetite in this way.

Reduces inflammation: Although the body naturally produces inflammation as a defense against injury or infection, persistent inflammation may result in a number of health issues, including obesity. The anti-inflammatory qualities of cayenne pepper's capsaicin may assist to lessen inflammation and enhance general health.

Enhances digestion: Cayenne pepper may improve digestion by stimulating the generation of digestive enzymes and boosting saliva production. This may facilitate better food digestion and lower the chance of digestive issues.

Cayenne pepper promotes perspiration and increases blood flow, which may assist the body cleanse by removing toxins and other toxic elements from the body.

Cayenne pepper may be a beneficial addition to a healthy diet and way of life for people aiming to reduce their weight and advance their general health and fitness. Before making any big changes to your food or fitness regimen, it's crucial to speak with a healthcare provider.

Sample meal plans and recipes:

Here are some sample meal plans and recipes to give you an idea of how you can incorporate healthy foods into your diet:

Meal Plan 1

Breakfast: Greek yogurt with mixed berries and a drizzle of honey
Snack: Apple slices with almond butter
Lunch: Grilled chicken breast with roasted sweet potatoes and green beans
Snack: Carrot sticks with hummus
Dinner: Baked salmon with asparagus and quinoa
Recipes

Greek Yogurt with Mixed Berries and Honey:

1 cup plain Greek yogurt
1/2 cup mixed berries
1 teaspoon honey
Mix the Greek yogurt with mixed berries in a bowl. Drizzle with honey and serve.

Grilled Chicken Breast with Roasted Sweet Potatoes and Green Beans:

1 boneless, skinless chicken breast
1 medium sweet potato, chopped
1 cup green beans
1 tablespoon olive oil
Salt and pepper to taste
Preheat the oven to 400°F. Toss the chopped sweet potato with olive oil, salt, and pepper. Roast in the oven for 20-25 minutes until tender.

Meanwhile, grill the chicken breast on a grill pan over medium-high heat until cooked through. Serve with steamed green beans.

Baked Salmon with Asparagus and Quinoa:

1 salmon fillet
1/2 bunch asparagus, trimmed
1/2 cup cooked quinoa
1 tablespoon olive oil
Salt and pepper to taste
Preheat the oven to 400°F. Place the salmon fillet in a baking dish and brush with olive oil. Season with salt and pepper. Bake for 15-20 minutes until cooked through. Meanwhile, roast the asparagus in the oven for 10-15 minutes until tender. Serve with cooked quinoa.

Meal Plan 2

Breakfast: Oatmeal with banana and walnuts
Snack: Celery sticks with cream cheese
Lunch: Turkey and avocado wrap with mixed greens
Snack: Hard boiled egg
Dinner: Vegetable stir-fry with brown rice
Recipes

Oatmeal with Banana and Walnuts:

1/2 cup rolled oats
1 cup water
1/2 banana, sliced
1 tablespoon chopped walnuts
Bring the water to a boil in a small saucepan. Add the oats and reduce the heat to low. Simmer for 5-10 minutes until thickened. Top

with banana slices and chopped walnuts.

Turkey and Avocado Wrap with Mixed Greens:

1 whole wheat wrap
2 slices turkey breast
1/2 avocado, sliced
1/4 cup mixed greens
1 tablespoon Dijon mustard
Spread the Dijon mustard on the wrap. Layer the turkey, avocado, and mixed greens on top. Roll up the wrap and serve.

Vegetable Stir-Fry with Brown Rice:

1 cup cooked brown rice
1/2 cup sliced bell pepper
1/2 cup sliced zucchini
1/2 cup sliced mushrooms
1 tablespoon soy sauce

1 tablespoon olive oil
Heat the olive oil in a large skillet over medium-high heat. Add the bell pepper, zucchini, and mushrooms. Stir-fry for 5-10 minutes until tender. Add the soy sauce and toss to combine. Serve with cooked brown rice.

CHAPTER THREE
Tips for Success on the Cayenne Pepper Diet.

The Cayenne Pepper Diet, sometimes called the Master Cleanse or Lemonade Diet, is a brief detoxification regimen that entails consuming a concoction of water, lemon juice, maple syrup, and cayenne pepper for a few days. The following advice will help you succeed with the cayenne pepper diet:

Consult your doctor: If you have any medical concerns or are already taking any drugs, it's crucial to speak with your doctor before beginning the cayenne pepper diet.

Be psychologically prepared: The Cayenne Pepper Diet may be difficult on both a physical and psychological level. Setting reasonable expectations and objectives for oneself, as well as cultivating a supportive environment, are crucial steps in mental preparation.

Drink lots of water to stay hydrated: Dehydration is a risk while following the Cayenne Pepper Diet. You should consume at least six to eight glasses of water daily in addition to the lemonade combination.

Take it easy: It's crucial to take it easy and avoid intense exercise when following the Cayenne Pepper Diet. You can feel tired or lightheaded, so it's crucial to pay attention to your body and take breaks as needed.

After finishing the Cayenne Pepper Diet, it's crucial to gently ease back into solid meals over the course of a few days. To gradually reintroduce additional foods, start with light, simple-to-digest items like fruits, vegetables, and soups.

Avoid alcohol and caffeine: It's crucial to stay away from alcohol and caffeine while on the Cayenne Pepper Diet since they may dehydrate the body and thwart the detoxification process.

The Cayenne Pepper Diet is not for everyone, therefore it's crucial to pay attention to your body and quit the diet if you start experiencing any unfavorable symptoms or health issues.

How to stay motivated on the Cayenne Pepper Diet:

The Cayenne Pepper Diet is a tough and restricted diet, making it difficult to stay motivated while following it. The following advice can help you remain motivated:

Realistic objectives are important to set since they may help you remain motivated. Focus on how the diet may enhance your general health and well-being rather than how many pounds you wish to reduce.

Keep a journal: Journaling may help you remain motivated and measure your progress. Think about how the diet is affecting your body and mind as you reflect on your thoughts, feelings, and experiences.

Find a support network: Having a network of people to turn to for support may keep you accountable and motivated. Find a buddy who is following the Cayenne Pepper Diet and join an online forum where you can discuss your successes and setbacks.

Focus on the advantages: Pay attention to the advantages of the diet rather than its drawbacks. You may improve your digestion, increase energy levels, and cleanse your body with the aid of the cayenne pepper diet.

The Cayenne Pepper Diet should be followed for a limited amount of time, thus it's crucial to take each day as it comes. Keep your attention on getting through each day, and celebrate each little triumph.

Reward yourself: Giving yourself a reward for sticking to your plan will keep you motivated. Give yourself a massage, a new outfit, or a fun night out with your friends.

Remain optimistic: Remaining optimistic might help you remain motivated and get over any challenges. To maintain your happy attitude, engage in gratitude exercises, affirmations, and visualization.

Coping with detox symptoms:

Dealing with detox symptoms .

It might be difficult to deal with detox symptoms, particularly in the early days of the Cayenne Pepper Diet. Following are some advice for managing withdrawal symptoms:

Water consumption is important since it helps your body remove toxins and eases detoxification symptoms. Along with the lemonade combination, try to have at least 6 to 8 glasses of water daily.

Get adequate sleep: Sleep is essential when on the cayenne pepper diet since it helps your body concentrate on cleansing. Make sure you get adequate rest, and if necessary, take naps or breaks throughout the day.

Deep breathing exercises will help you relax and lessen the effects of detoxification. Try inhaling deeply through your nose and expelling through your mouth while breathing slowly.

Use herbal remedies: Ginger, chamomile, and peppermint are a few examples of herbs that might aid with nausea and other detox symptoms. Try taking herbal pills or sipping herbal tea.

Take a warm bath: A warm bath may soothe you and aid with detoxification symptoms. If you want to maximize the advantages of your bath, add Epsom salt or aromatic fragrances like lavender.

Engage in light exercise: Activities like yoga, walking, or stretching may promote circulation, lymphatic system stimulation, and detox symptoms. Avoid physically demanding activities or those that might drain your energy.

If necessary, get medical attention if you develop severe or lingering withdrawal symptoms. Your doctor can assist you in determining if the symptoms are caused by the cayenne pepper diet or whether another underlying problem requires treatment.

CHAPTER FOUR:
Safety and precautions.

You may safely and effectively cleanse your body with the cayenne pepper diet, but there are several safety and well-being measures you should take beforehand. Here are some crucial safety and preventative steps to think about:

Before beginning the program, speak with your doctor, particularly if you have any health issues or are on any drugs.

Never stick to the diet for longer than the suggested 10-day period. Longer-term diet adherence might result in vitamin shortages and other health issues.

To flush out toxins and avoid being dehydrated, drink lots of water.

Avoid physically demanding activities or those that might drain your energy.

Seek medical attention if your withdrawal symptoms are severe or prolonged.

Once the diet is over, slowly introduce solid food back into your diet. To gradually reintroduce additional foods, start with light, simple-to-digest items like fruits, vegetables, and soups.

Avoid drinking and using caffeine during and after the diet since they might cause your body to become dehydrated and interfere with the detoxification process.

Use the diet just temporarily to lose weight. The Cayenne Pepper Diet is intended for quick detoxification; it is not recommended for long-term weight reduction.

If you are under 18 years old, pregnant, or breastfeeding, do not follow the diet.

People with specific medical issues, such as diabetes, eating disorders, liver or renal illness, or digestive difficulties, should not follow the cayenne pepper diet. Before beginning the program, discuss any underlying medical issues you may have with your healthcare physician.

Frequently Asked Questions about the Cayenne Pepper Diet:

What is the Cayenne Pepper Diet?
The Cayenne Pepper Diet, also known as the Master Cleanse or Lemonade Diet, is a short-term detox diet that involves drinking a mixture of lemon juice, maple syrup, cayenne pepper, and water for several days to cleanse the body of toxins.

How long does the Cayenne Pepper Diet last?
The Cayenne Pepper Diet typically lasts for 10 days, although some people may choose to do it for shorter or longer periods of time. It

is not recommended to do the diet for more than 10 days at a time.

What are the benefits of the Cayenne Pepper Diet?
The Cayenne Pepper Diet is believed to have several benefits, including weight loss, improved digestion, increased energy, and a reduction in inflammation. However, there is limited scientific evidence to support these claims.

Is the Cayenne Pepper Diet safe?
The Cayenne Pepper Diet can be safe for most people when done correctly and for a short period of time. However, it is not recommended for people with certain medical conditions, such as diabetes, kidney disease, or heart problems. It is also important

to consult with a healthcare provider before starting the diet.

Can you eat while on the Cayenne Pepper Diet?
No, the Cayenne Pepper Diet involves consuming only the lemon juice, maple syrup, cayenne pepper, and water mixture for the duration of the diet. Solid food is not allowed.

Will the Cayenne Pepper Diet help me lose weight?
The Cayenne Pepper Diet may help you lose weight in the short term due to the low calorie intake. However, any weight loss is likely to be temporary, as it is primarily due to water loss and not fat loss. It is not recommended as a long-term weight loss solution.

How do I prepare the Cayenne Pepper Diet drink?

To prepare the Cayenne Pepper Diet drink, mix 2 tablespoons of freshly squeezed lemon juice, 2 tablespoons of maple syrup, 1/10 teaspoon of cayenne pepper, and 8-10 ounces of water. Drink this mixture 6-12 times per day for the duration of the diet.

Can I exercise while on the Cayenne Pepper Diet?

Light exercise, such as walking or yoga, is usually allowed while on the Cayenne Pepper Diet. However, it is important to listen to your body and avoid strenuous exercise while on a low-calorie diet.

What should I do after completing the Cayenne Pepper Diet?

After completing the Cayenne Pepper Diet, it is important to ease back into a normal, healthy diet gradually. Start by consuming light, easily digestible foods and gradually reintroduce solid foods over several days. It is also important to drink plenty of water to rehydrate the body.

Exploring alternative approaches:

Certainly! The Cayenne Pepper Diet may not be the greatest choice for everyone since there are many alternative ways to have a healthy physique. Here are some other strategies you could think about investigating:

Eating a balanced diet is one of the most important methods to maintain excellent health. A balanced diet should contain a range of nutrient-dense foods. Consume more entire foods, such as fresh produce, whole grains, lean meats, and healthy fats.

Restricting food intake for a certain amount of time each day or week is known as intermittent fasting. Intermittent fasting can help with weight loss and enhance metabolic health. There are many different ways to do it.

Mindful eating entails focusing on the food you consume and being in the present moment while you eat. This may improve your food choices, increase meal enjoyment, and decrease overeating.

Eating foods that support your liver and kidneys will aid in your body's natural detoxification process. Leafy greens, beets, garlic, turmeric, and ginger are a few examples.

Exercise on a regular basis is essential for keeping excellent health. Find a hobby you love and make an effort to exercise for at least 30 minutes most days of the week.

Always pay attention to your body's signals and choose a strategy that works for you. For advice on what could be the best course of action for you, speak with a certified dietitian or healthcare professional.